Using an X-Acto knife, a single sheet of paper, and the inspiration that surrounds her at her Olympia, Washington, home, Nikki McClure lovingly creates her intricate and beautiful paper cuts. Her work constructs a bold graphic language that embraces motherhood, nature, and activism. Nikki makes books, journals, and a yearly calendar when she is not picking berries with her family.

www.nikkimcclure.com

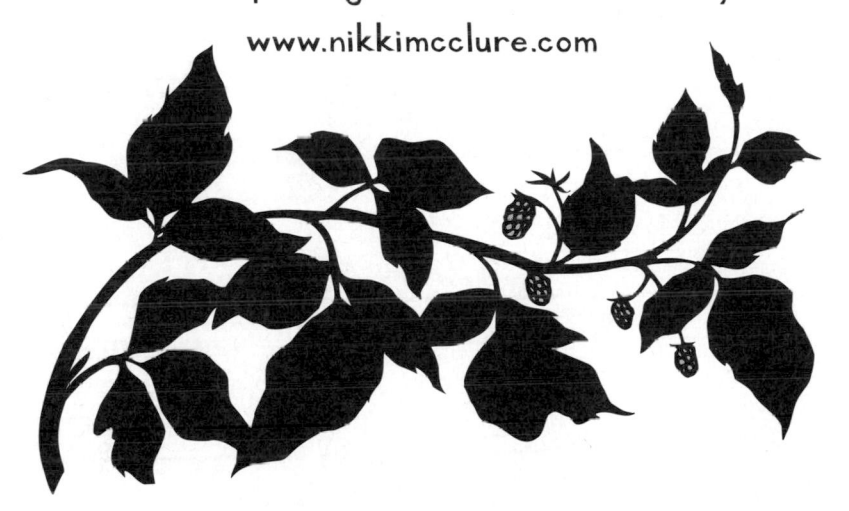

Printed in China
Printed on recycled paper
Published by Sasquatch Books
Distributed by PGW/Perseus

17 16 15 14 13 12 11   9 8 7 6 5 4 3 2 1

Book design: Kate Basart/Union Pageworks

ISBN-13: 978-1-57061-681-5   ISBN-10: 1-57061-681-7

SASQUATCH BOOKS
et, Suite 400, Seattle, WA 98104 | 206.467.4300
books.com | custserv@sasquatchbooks.com

HELPERS

Who can I call on for help?

cleaning

making food

grocery shopping

breast-feeding

a hug when I am overwhelmed

RESOURCES IN MY COMMUNITY

people and places to turn to for assistance

_____

_____

_____

_____

_____

_____

_____

_____

_____

_____

_____

_____

_____

_____

go on one last date

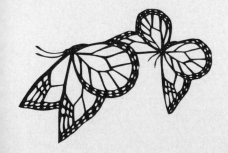

last day of work!

massage, ultrasound

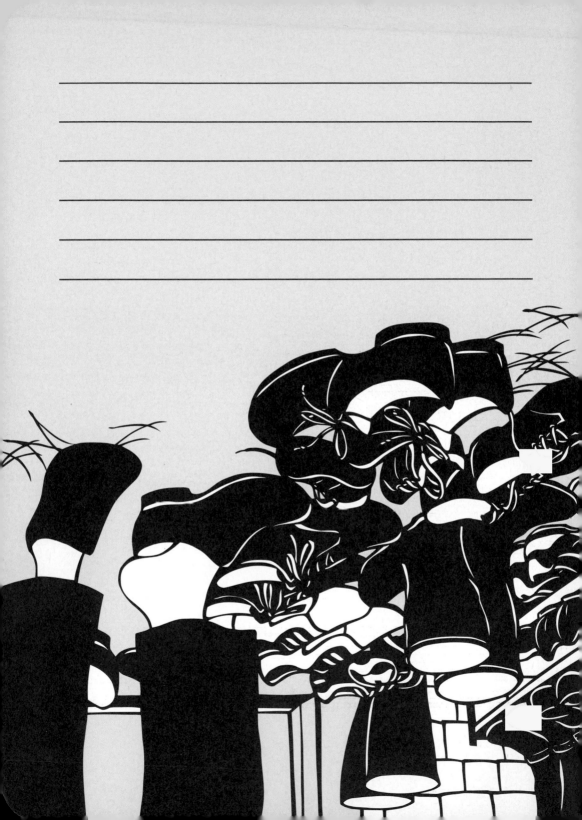

APPOINTMENTS

doctor, midwife

_____

_____

_____

_____

_____

_____

_____

_____

_____

_____

_____

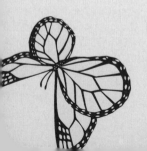

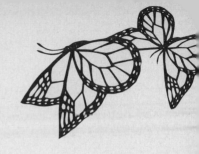

Not these ones!

old family names

NAMES

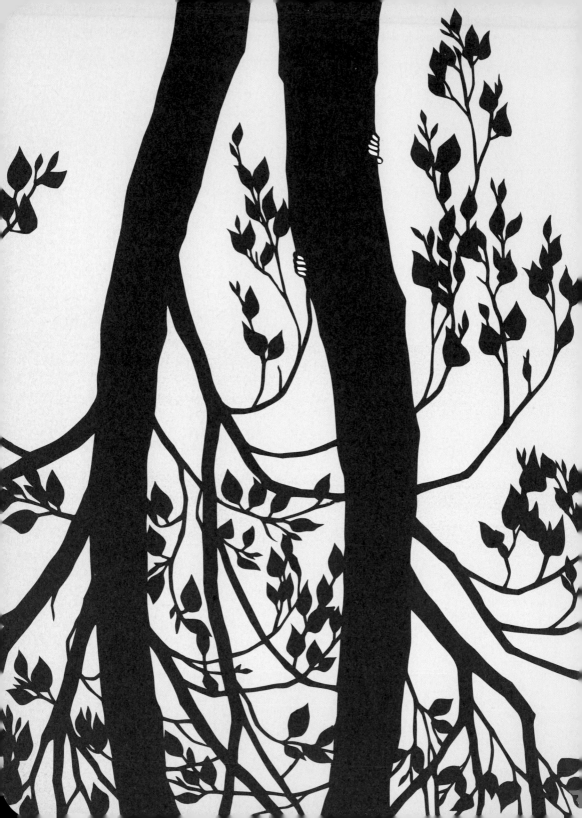

Love. Love. Love.

offers of help

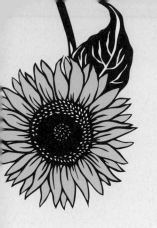

Who takes care of my family?

Who takes care of me?

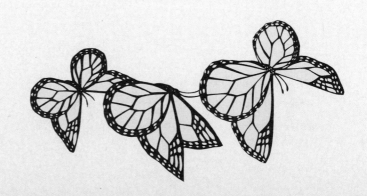

NURTURE

how I take care of myself and my baby

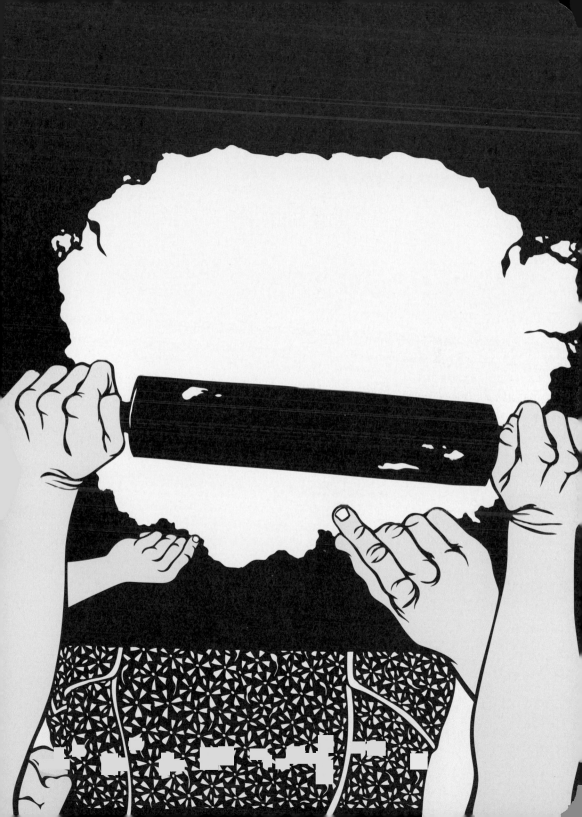

score cookies from the café

the whole town

children

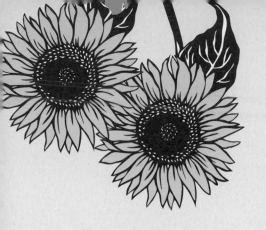

friends

brothers

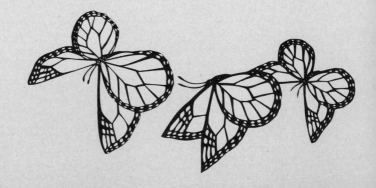

sisters

wishes from fathers

wishes from mothers

WELCOME

wishes of love for me and my baby

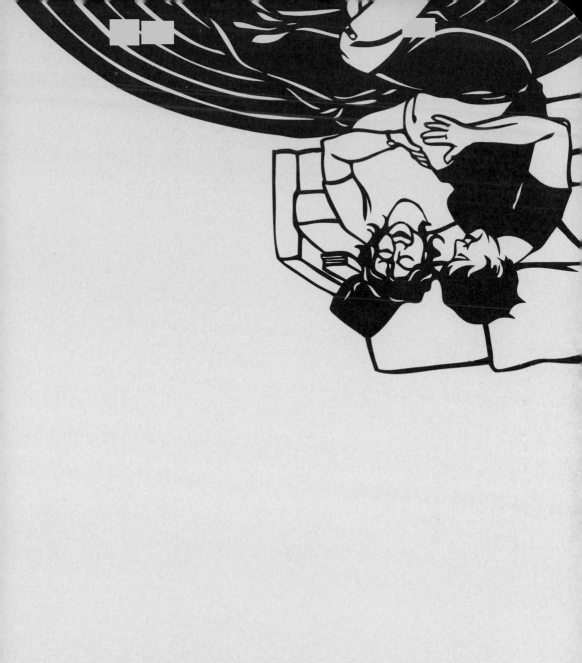

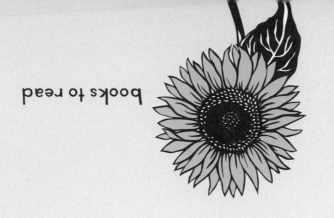

books to read

gathering courage

emotional changes

TRANSFORM

photos and drawings of my changing body

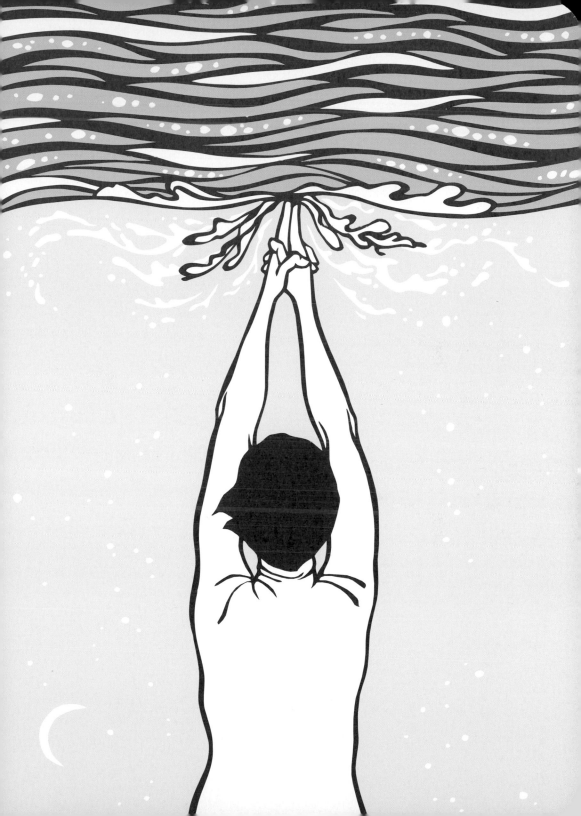

crazy nesting plans

make baby's bookshelf

Who wants to make us dinner?

Who will spread the news?

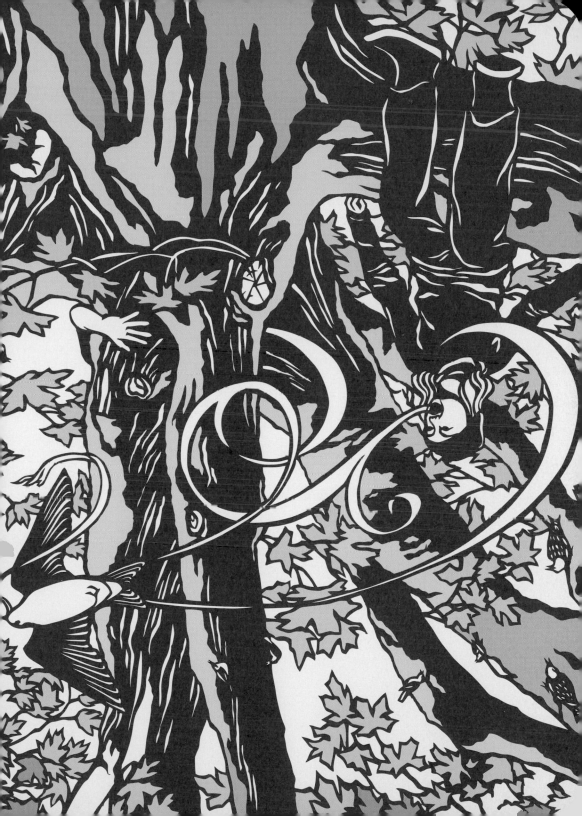

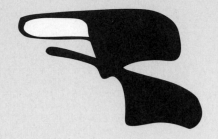

HOSPITAL BAG

robe, slippers, snacks, camera, music

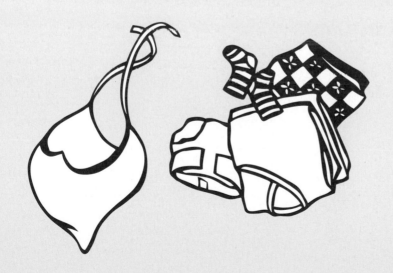

Homemade Wipe Recipe

  1½ cups water

  1 tablespoon almond or jojoba oil

  1 tablespoon baby soap (like Dr. Bronner's mild)

  1 to 2 drops tea tree oil

Mix everything in large bucket with secure lid.

Cut paper towel roll in half along the middle with a sharp, non-serrated knife, removing the cardboard tube from center. Stand one half of the paper towel roll in bucket with uncut side down. Let it soak for a few minutes and flip so cut side is down. Put lid on until ready to use.

When using wipes, pull from center of roll. If you are going away for a few days, place wipes in fridge so they don't get moldy. You can also add a few drops of essential oils if you wish.

Fill a small zip-top baggie for the diaper bag. Easy!

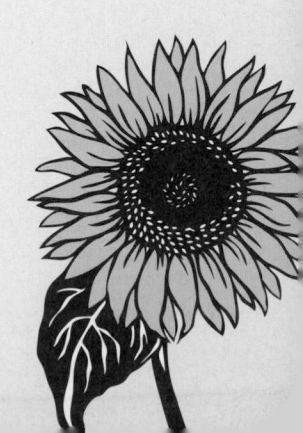

all you really need are diapers
and a changing pad

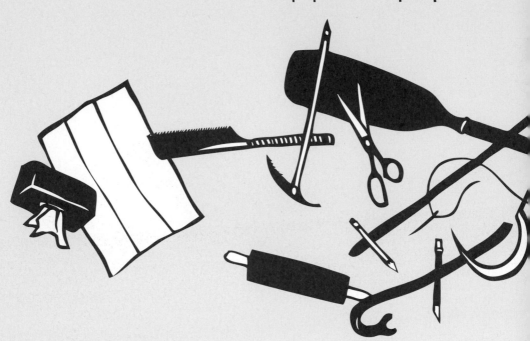

birthing supply list

PREPARE

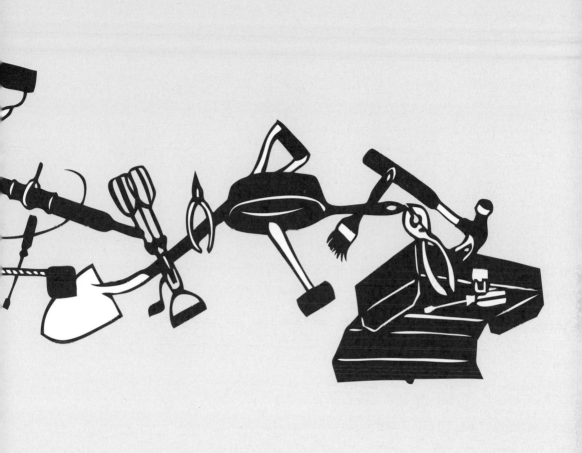

hopes for my family

hopes for me as a mother

wishes for the birth

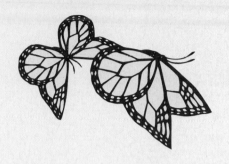

dreams of courage and trust

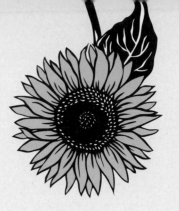

dreams of change

dreams of the baby

DREAMS

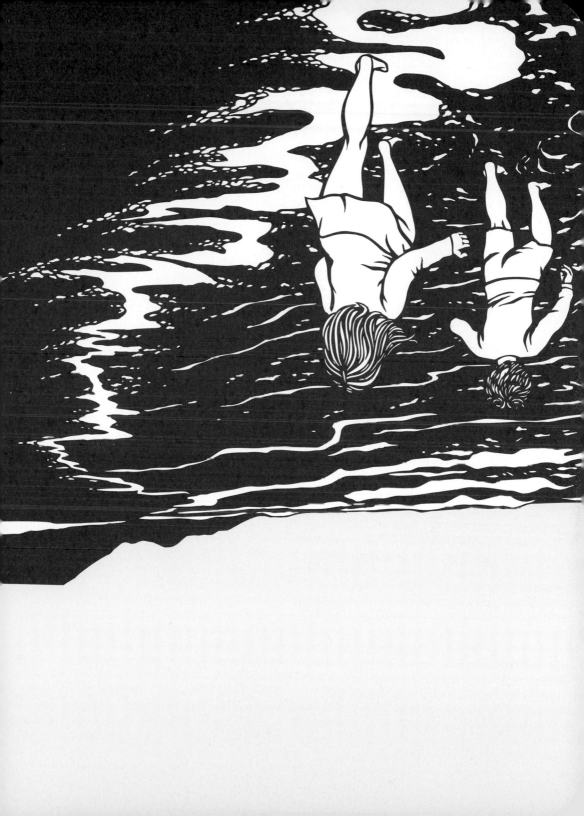

welcomes from far away

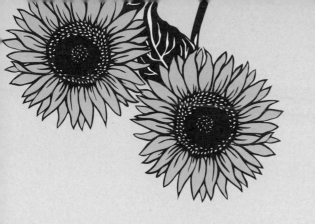

first visitors

settling in

the excitement and peace of our new family

first yawn, first nap, first sight of each other

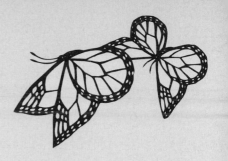

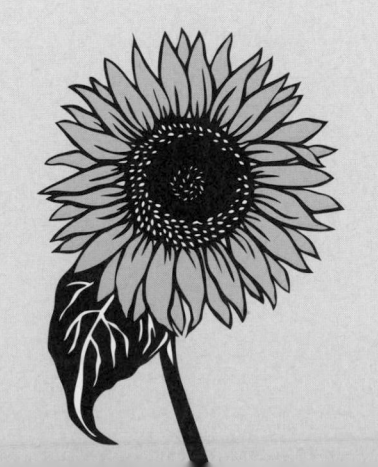

nursing and nuzzling

surrender

I am a Mother.

my baby!

my birthing story

10th MONTH

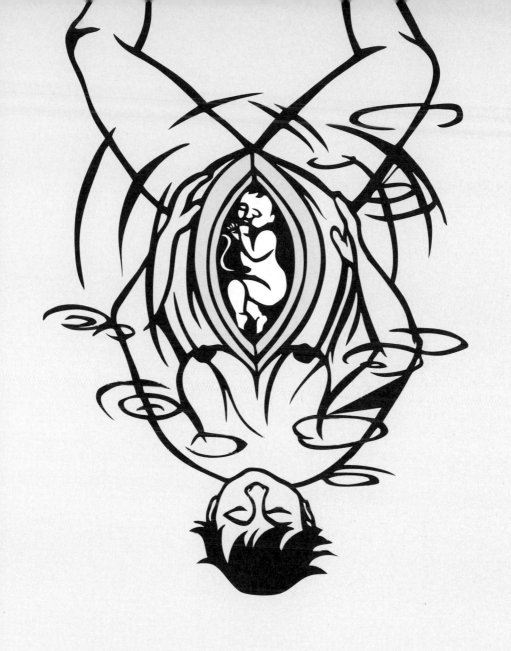

the summoning, the call to begin

WAYS TO PASS THE TIME

start a quilt that will never be finished

rest!

climb a mountain

clean out the refrigerator

talk to friends for hours

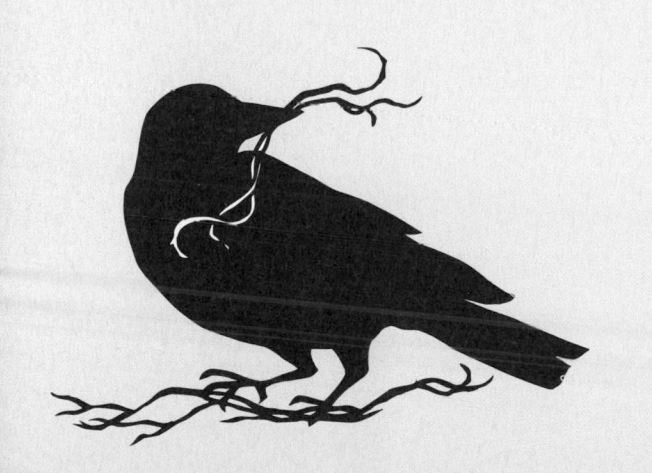

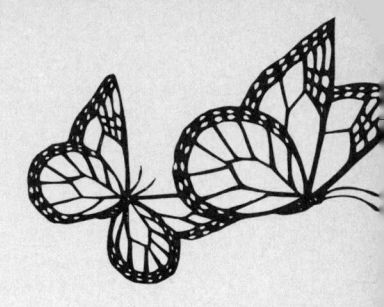

drawing of baby ready inside

drawing of my belly button

nesting, preparing the burrow

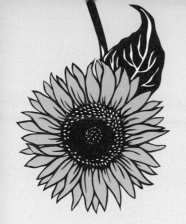

my birth plan

waiting

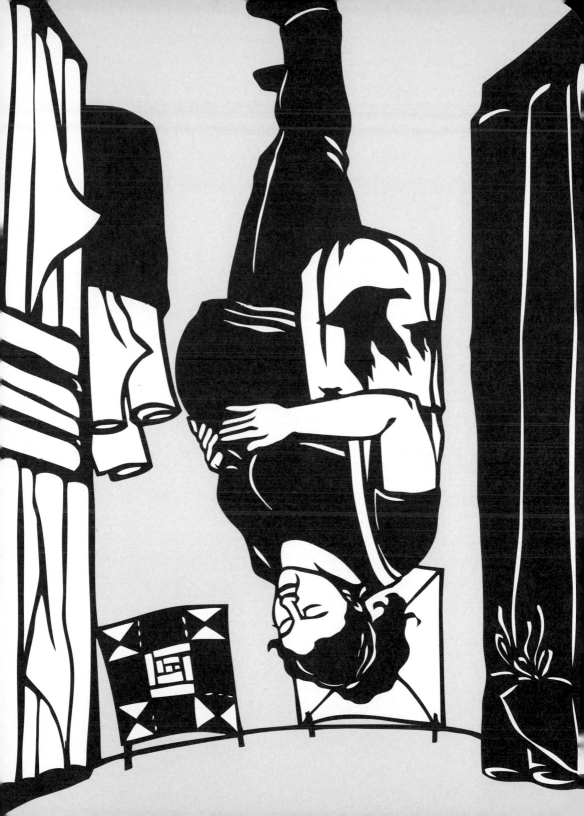

ADVICE FROM STRANGERS

ADVICE FROM FRIENDS

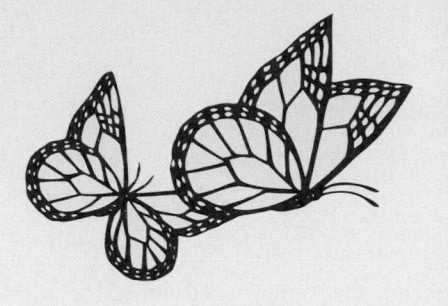

return library books

get a car seat ready

for every day past your due date,
    do something nice for yourself

searching for my baby's doctor

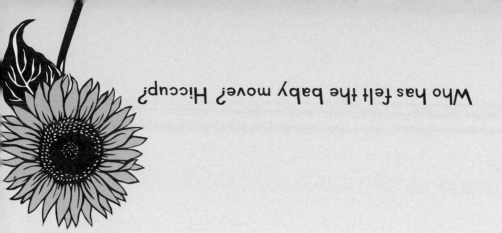

Who has felt the baby move? Hiccup?

and all those good wishes

baby shower plans

8th MONTH

I am so pregnant.

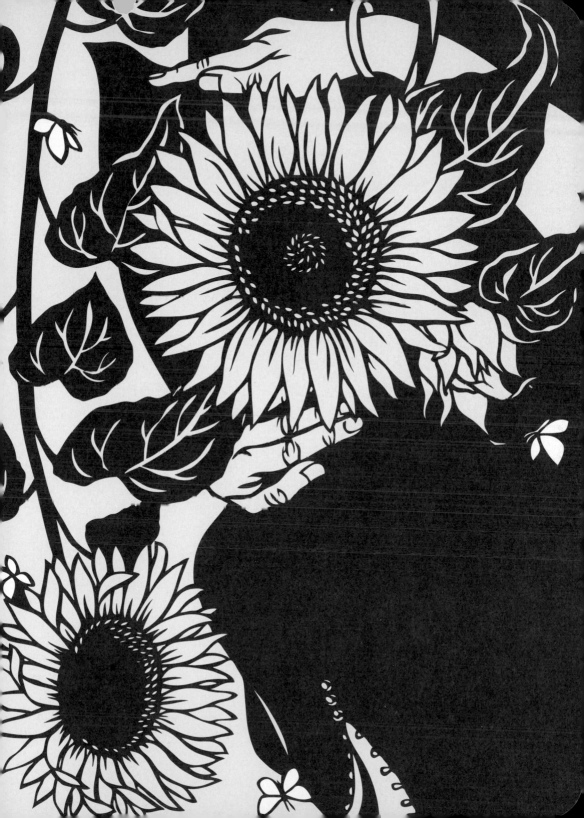

go for a long walk and take a long nap

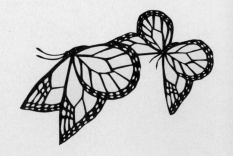

see a movie

make a movie

especially my own

talk to other mothers

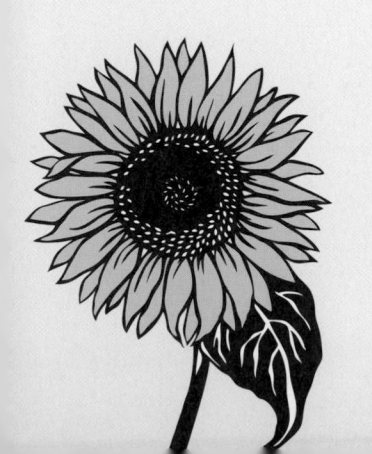

Birth class? Massage?

Diaper service? Freeze a lasagna?

7th MONTH

Get things done!

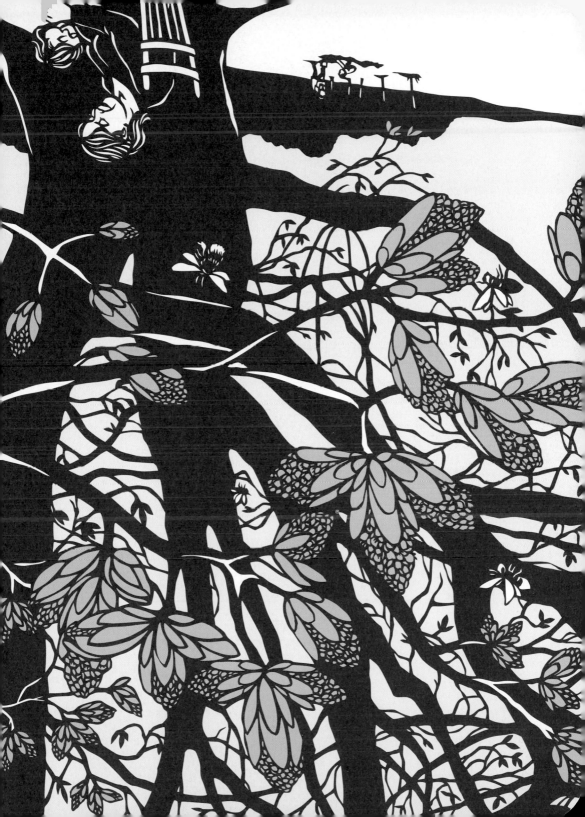

grow, grow, grow, and drink nettle tea

   crumble dried nettles and mint leaves into teapot,
   add hot water,
   steep for five minutes,
   pour and add honey

One last getaway trip?
a babymoon

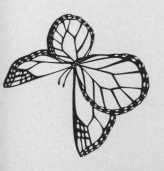

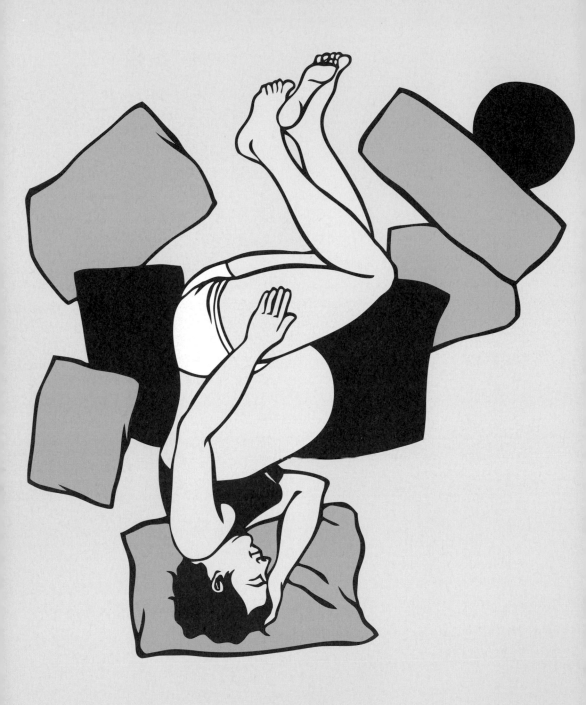

my pillow arrangement

What was I like as a baby?

What was my mother like?

What kind of mother will I be?

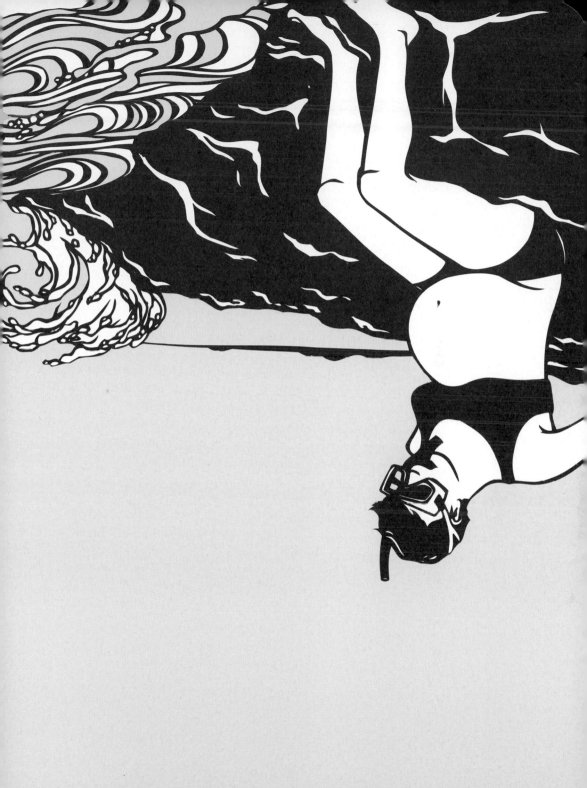

I am confident and beautiful.

my favorite snacks

foot rubs, friends, naps, more food

new aches and cramps

your nose, fingers, feet

I can see you.

ultrasound images

5th MONTH

gravity is shifting

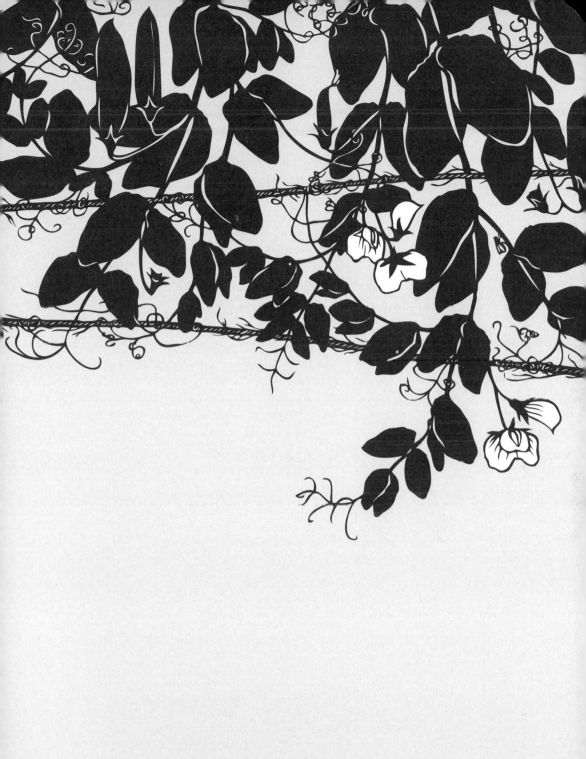

feelings about my family

deepening connection to my partner
and support from my community

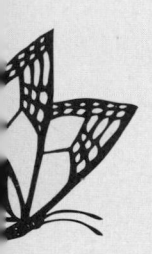

feeling my baby fluttering inside

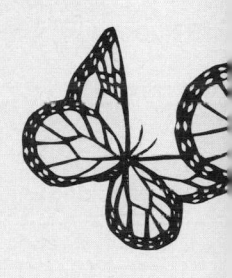

my belly cannot be contained

rubber bands hold my pants on
    for one more week

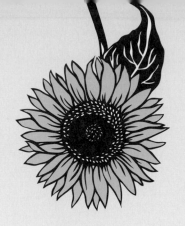

glow, love, smile all day

my energy returns, yoga, walk, swim

this is really happening

4th MONTH

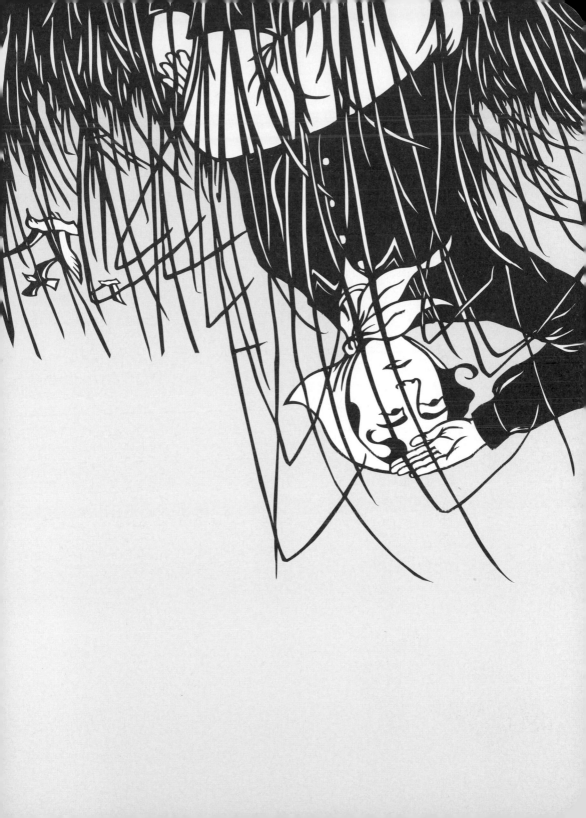

accepting and growing

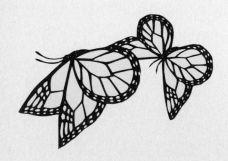

celebrating this new life inside me

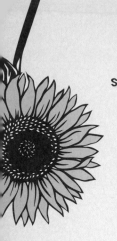

sharing the news

shouting it out to the world

love the love

how tired I am

3rd MONTH

Am I showing?

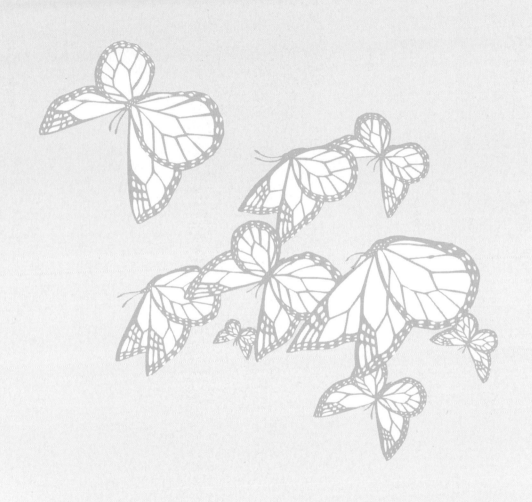

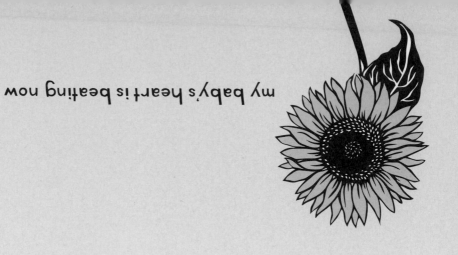

my baby's heart is beating now

good food to grow a strong baby

searching for a midwife or doctor

taking care of myself

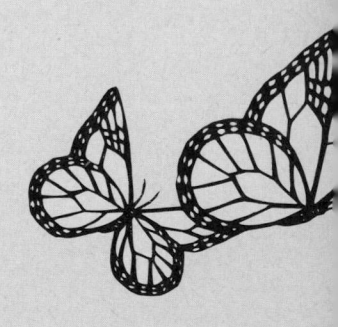

things that make me queasy

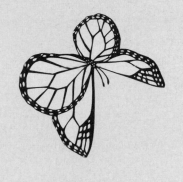

what I crave

sharing my body is work

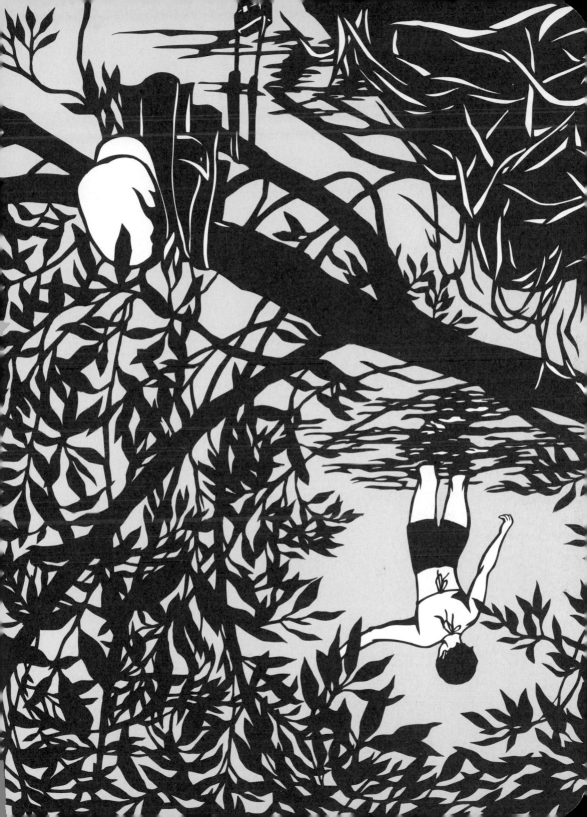

take a walk with my best friend

special places to rest at home and work

I am pregnant!!!!!

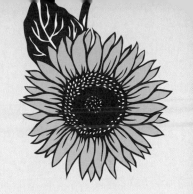

Who have I told this secret to?

My breasts are so big!

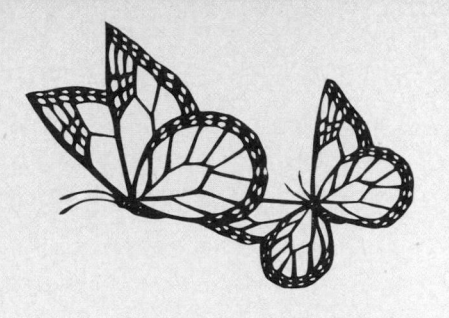

I am pregnant. I am pregnant. I am pregnant.

it is all I can think of

GROW

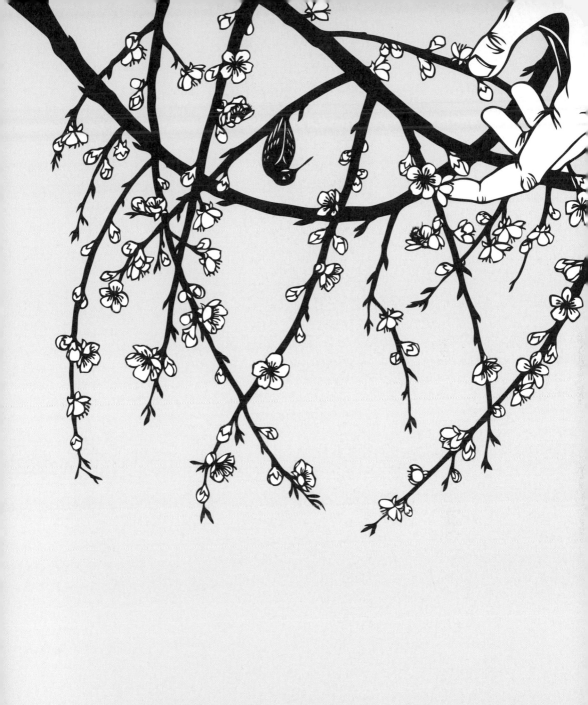

laughing, thinking, embracing

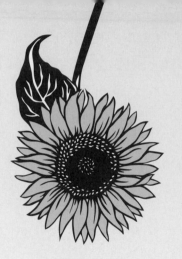

excitement, worry, joy, fear

EMBRACE

preparing for this new adventure

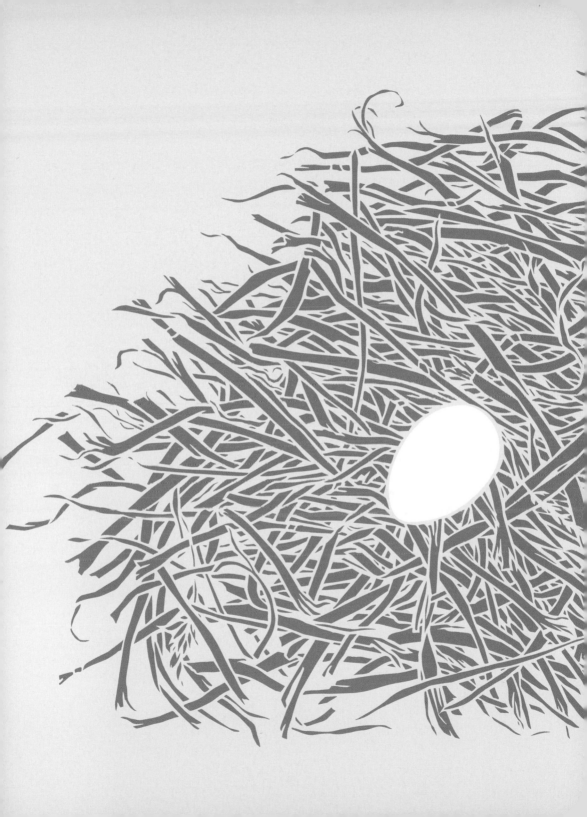

telling my partner

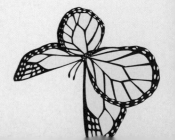

early inklings of this baby inside

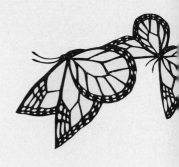

how I knew I was pregnant

DISCOVER

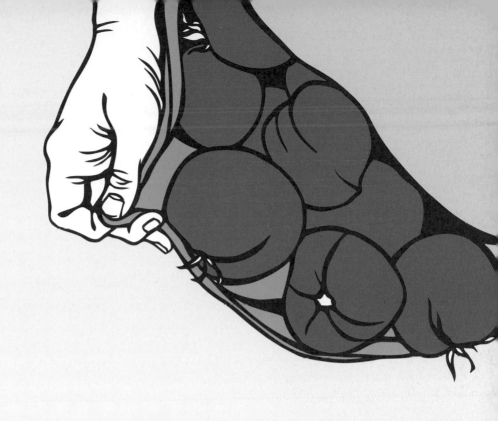

the searching

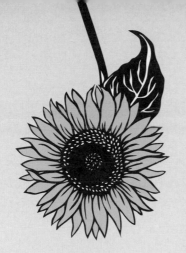

the yearning

DESIRE

how I wanted a baby

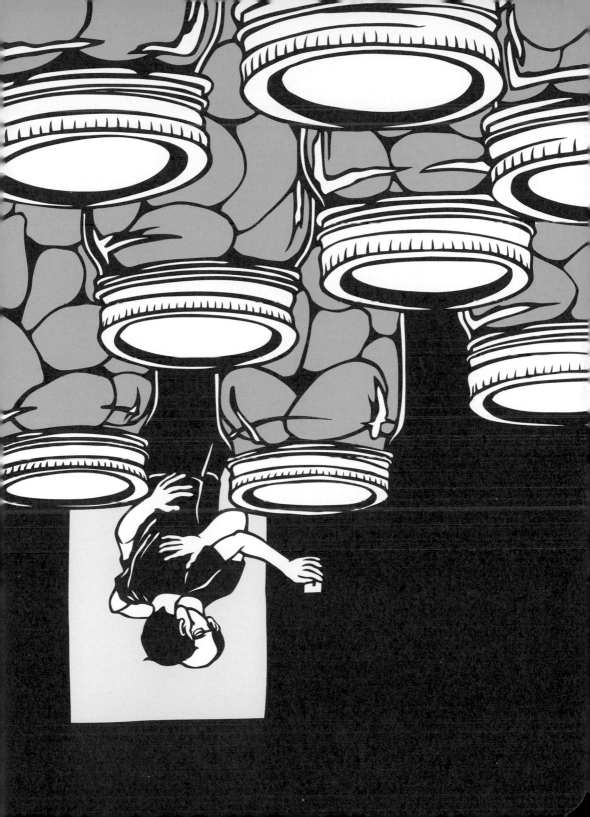

SASQUATCH BOOKS
SEATTLE

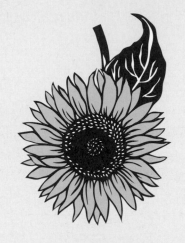

Nikki McClure

EMBRACE
A Pregnancy Journal

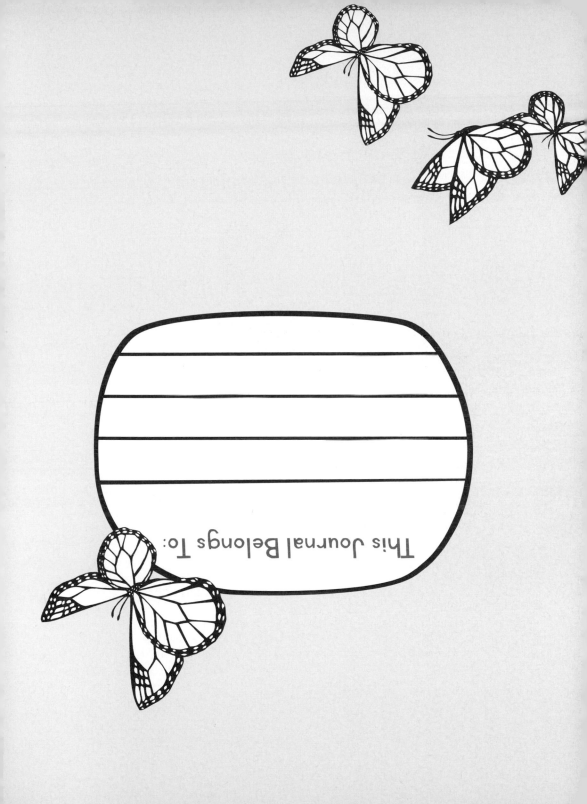

This Journal Belongs To:

EMBRACE